Cut, Cool, and Confident:

How to get rid of Beer Belly, Chicken Legs, Wimp Arms, and Man Boobs. And much, much more!

By

Jack Witt

With illustrations by

Kaitlin Howell

2

Table of Contents

Part I

Part II

Part III

Introduction

Today we live in a very fast-paced, technologically advanced, rapid-fire Information Age. It's hard to find time for oneself and close friends and family, let alone get to the gym for a workout and cook a healthy meal afterwards. The workweek and commute times are getting longer, and it seems like social networking is eating up a lot of our time, creating empty connections and unnecessary distractions. Add this all together, and you get lots of barriers to health and wellness that we must acknowledge and overcome.

In this book I try to turn back the clock to a simpler, more innocent time with retro- looking, 1950's/1960's illustrations, humorous anecdotes and a light-hearted atmosphere regarding exercise, nutrition and motivation. It's my aim to harness everything I've learned in my ten years as a health and fitness coach to people of all ages, sizes, and personalities, and to create some simple steps and techniques to help you understand and take charge of your health and well being, while having fun doing it!

I've always felt that fitness and health doesn't have to be overly serious, it doesn't have to be complicated and tedious; it can be a part of your life, not consuming your life. I'm not a super athletic person naturally (I've had to develop that), and when I was growing up in school I was a bit of a class clown, more into music and being in a rock band than playing sports and being a popular jock.

That said, o-happy days are here again, folks, and I'm gonna "sock it to you" with unique and uncomplicated methods for keeping yourself motivated and "bird is the word" on how your food management doesn't have to be rocket science. You'll get some very specific exercise instructions on how to get rid of those "radioactive" common problem areas on the human body, and you'll look and feel terrific as a result!

So enjoy my companion books; *"Tight, Tone & Trim: How to get rid of Cankles, Bat Wings, Thunder Thighs, & Muffin Tops"* and *"Cut, Cool & Confident: How to get rid of Beer Belly, Chicken Legs, Wimp Arms, & Man Boobs"*. E-book versions featuring full color illustrations are available at https://www.amazon.com/author/jackwitt at a discounted price.

Cheers,

Jack Witt
Health and Fitness Coach

SMEFADSAI

I proclaim today as the first day of the rest of your life! Roll out the banners, ticker tape, and marching bands because you are on your way to a brighter tomorrow. You know life is short and it goes by quickly. You know it's never too late to change. You know you have so much untapped potential inside of you.

So today I want you to make a pact with yourself that there's no more looking back, no more being stuck in the present and staring at that face and that body in the mirror, that you simply are not connecting with. I'm yelling at you now, at the top of my lungs, so your inner child baby thing can hear me, "Hey, Real You! Yeah, YOU, way deep down inside, buried and smooshed underneath the façade of this person with Beer Belly, Chicken Legs, Wimp Arms, and Man Boobs, it's time to take charge of your fitness, health, and wellness and discover a whole new world of possibilities!"

I truly want you to look your best and be CUT, COOL, and CONFIDENT! It's not going to be easy, and there are going to be days where you want to throw in the towel and go back to being the old you that you've grown comfortable with. But I'm sayin' stick with me, folks, 'cause I'm going to show you and I'm going to tell you how to be a fit, happy, and healthy person.

Can you feel it? I call this the process and journey to getting Cut, Cool, and Confident…(sound of a record scratching and/or crickets chirping) "?" Wait a minute; actually, I don't have a special homeopathic, rhyming, or spiritual sounding name for it. So, uh, let's just call it "Stop Making Excuses, Focus, and Do Something About It!" or SMEFADSAI for short.

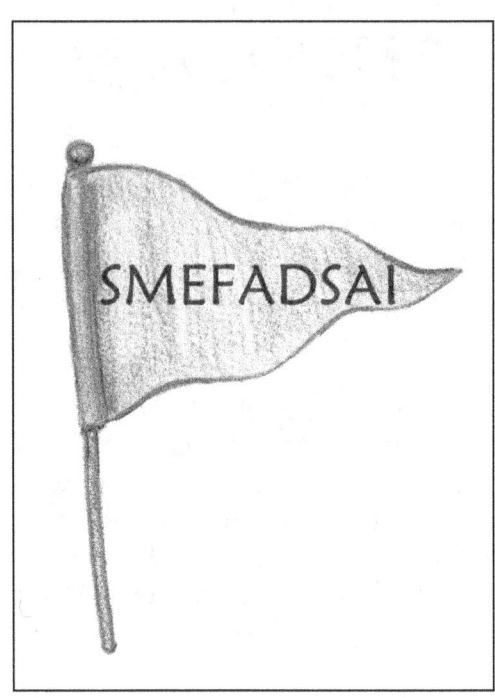

In all my years in the health and fitness industry, helping people of all ages, shapes, and sizes, there are a few common traits or mindsets that I've discovered the most successful clients harness on their journey to a successful SMEFADSAI.

Emotional Intelligence

The first SMEFADSAI is going to be tuning up your emotional intelligence. I live in Hollywood, or, "Hollyweird," as it is sometimes called. Everything here in Tinsel Town revolves around the motion picture industry. It's lights, camera, and action here every day, 24/7. So, I liken emotional intelligence to having the ability to stop the movie that is YOU in your life, step outside of the frame as the actor, YOU, look back at yourself now, as YOU, the director, by slowing the movie frames down and taking notice of how you act and react to certain situations and happenings in your day-to-day life.

In particular, and very importantly, is how you deal with your stressors. Too much stress all at once, or cumulatively over a long period of time, combined with not so good coping habits, can cause chemical, physical, and even hormonal imbalances in your body. These imbalances can lead to all kinds of problems like being overweight, obesity, suppressed immune functions, cancer, high blood pressure, heart attacks, stroke, and death if left unchecked.

Every stressor that we have usually causes a bad habit if not properly dealt with. Some people stress and then eat sweets or salty foods. Some people stress and zone out and watch TV. Whatever it is, take a look at the character of you in your life movie and observe, take notes, and assess how you react and behave in certain situations. Do you like what you are seeing? Or, can you re-write the script to your movie and feature the character of YOU managing stressors better and living a healthier, fit and fulfilled life? This ability is crucial in making the first step towards positive change. Once you make those changes, the Oscar goes to you! (We know; you'd like to thank all the little people!)

It typically takes about 30 to 45 days of consistency to break a bad habit and/or get into a good habit. So I want you to identify a behavior, action, or habit from your life movie that you want to manage first and set up a 30-day action plan to success. Here's how it works: Each day you will do something to counteract that bad habit and/or bring about positive change in your life. For instance, if you come home from work and immediately turn on the TV and zone out with munchies or alcoholic drinks, your 30-day action plan might feature you coming home from work and simply deep breathing for 20 minutes, then stretching for 10 minutes, before you allow yourself to turn on the TV.

Do this for 30 days straight to bring about change. The great thing is, it's like a domino effect - once you break one bad habit there are positive lifestyle changes that will happen in several other areas in your life as a result. How cool is that? You do one positive thing, and a bunch of other little positive things will start happening. You can email me at Jack@GetFitwithWitt.com for a free action plan template. Trust yourself and enjoy your voyage of discovery to a better you.

Faith in Fitness

Another SMEFADSAI is simply having faith in fitness. Can I get a witness?! And it's really more about having faith in the process of fitness and health. You might have faith in God, faith in a person in your life or your family, faith in your community and/or government (well, maybe not government, huh). So you must develop faith in how making positive, healthy changes in your life will help your body, mind, spirit, career, relationships, and circle of family and friends.

I mean, think about it. Have you really ever heard of anybody praising the virtues of being unhealthy and how being unhealthy has helped them with anything in their lives? Well, having faith in fitness and health really isn't taking a big risk. I personally guarantee you that good things will come from it, if you stick to it and make it part of your lifestyle. You've got to have faith! Believe in yourself and who you can become, because if you don't nobody else will.

Get a Little Crazy

Another SMEFADSAI is that you just have to get a little crazy! Yeah, that's right - wacky, insane, and wildly weird about exercise and eating well. As adults we may have a tendency to over think things, dwell on the past, beat ourselves up, or worry about the future. To an extent we must do those things to be realistic about where we're going and what we're doing in our lives

But give yourself permission to just let loose when it comes to your health (in a positive way). Don't expect or demand instant results when starting an exercise program or improving your food intake. Don't dwell on what you are giving up (time and/or money). Don't even worry about what other people think. Just be crazy by trusting and embracing the process, which in turn will stir around those positive brain chemicals called endorphins that will be dancing and prancing around from your healthy and active lifestyle, and in turn will get you "in the zone" of doing the right thing for your body and your mind.

You'll start to hit a stride, and the physically, mentally, and emotionally positive results will start to trickle in and culminate. You'll begin to have extra energy, extra focus and clarity, extra strength, flexibility and range of motion, to get through the normal challenges and obstacles of everyday life. Then the cosmetic changes will start happening and your body will start taking shape, just the way you want it. But notice, I said all this good stuff would start "trickling" in. This isn't a miracle pill or a potion, or a 7-steps-to-change-your-life-in-a-week type of scam. It's a one-day-at-a-time type of "inch-by-inch" approach that is realistic for an everyday, average person like me, and you, and it stays true to your human body, mind, and soul.

Each day will build on the last. Each positive change will snowball into several other positive changes, and a solid foundation will be laid for you to construct yourself into exactly what and who you have always wanted to be. You can't build a house overnight and expect it to be solid, strong, and last a long time. You have to lay the foundation brick by brick. I promise being a little crazy about health and fitness during the process of building YOU day by day does truly work! It might take longer than you want, or it might come sooner than you are ready for. Think about that one…Deep, ay?

Create a Support Network

The last SMEFADSAI is to create a network of support and throw the message out to the Universe every single day that you are adopting a healthier lifestyle and developing into the true you. I'm not talking New Year's Eve, early-January-type resolutions of, "I'm going to get in shape this year," when a few weeks into February all of your health and fitness goals are forgotten. I'm talking true commitment, a whatever-it-takes type of attitude, "This is do or die."

Find family members, and co-workers and friends with whom you can talk to, Facebook, text, tweet, Google Talk, instant message, or Skype (I'm trying to sound tech-savvy here, folks, but half of these will probably be obsolete by the time you read this book) with about what you are doing for your health each day. We all need support and encouragement when getting out of our comfort zone and trying to make positive changes. So use your sphere of influence and your connections to keep you motivated and focused.

You have to throw it out to the Universe each day that you are going to do, or have done, something positive for your body and mind during your transition. No matter how big or small, just keep throwing it out there and throwing it out there. We all know the story of "The Secret" - the Universe will provide back to you; it will supply you with somebody or something that will come into your life to propel and catapult you even further into good fitness, health and wellness. Whatever it turns out to be, embrace it and go with it. You are going to be a different person!

You know, being unhealthy and out of tune with your mind and body is sort of like the flip side of having an addiction problem. People who have addictions will lie, cheat, deceive and steal to keep their habit alive. It's usually not until they have some type of spiritual awakening, or commit to a lifestyle change program, treatment or therapy, that they finally overcome the problem.

Similarly, people who want to take charge of their health and fitness have to treat that process with the same sense of urgency and respect as those trying to shake an addiction. It's a sort of parallel universe; you are actually addicted to non-action, procrastination, fear and neglect of your mind, body, and spirit. I'm coining a new term for this: "Unhealthy-o-holic." So if you can hire a life coach, personal trainer, or professional therapist, do it and do it now!

Time to Get Started

Okay, guys (and maybe ladies if you are reading this), the next section of this book is dedicated to controlling those problem areas of your body: *Beer Belly, Chicken Legs, Wimp Arms, and Man Boobs.* Concentrate first on the most severe area of your body, and prioritize the rest from there. In addition to the directions and exercise plans I'll be laying out for you, you should also be doing some type of cardio every other day. This will not only help your heart become stronger and more efficient at pumping blood and oxygen throughout your body, but it will help with overall fat loss throughout your body, including those problem areas. Also, cardio really helps to kick up positive brain chemicals called endorphins, so you become mentally stronger and better able to overcome daily obstacles and life challenges. I would recommend at least 30 minutes per day of some type of cardio training. This could be anything from jogging, stationary bike, elliptical, and hiking, to running in place. If you are not sweating and a little out of breath, you are probably performing below the optimal level to create a fitness change. So, make sure your intensity is sufficient, and when 30 minutes starts to feel too easy, increase your time/duration and/or your intensity (i.e. incline on the treadmill, level of difficulty of your hike).

In addition to the directions and exercise plans I'll be laying out for you, you will need to also be doing some type of cardio every other day. This will help with general fat loss throughout your body, including those problem areas. I would recommend at least 30 minutes per day of some type of cardio training. This could be anything from jogging, stationary bike, elliptical, and hiking, to running in place. If you are not sweating and a little out of breath, you are probably performing below the optimal level to create a fitness change. So, make sure your intensity is sufficient, and when 30 minutes starts to feel too easy, increase your time/duration and/or your intensity (i.e. incline on the treadmill, level of difficulty of your hike).

One important rule to remember is how to calculate your maximum heart rate for safety purposes. That formula is 220-your age. For instance, if you are 40 years old, 220-40 = 180, so 180 heartbeats per minute is the upper level of where you should be. If it's anything over this number, you may be doing too much and need to slow down and lessen your time or intensity. Ideally, you should be at about 80% of this number (180 x 80% = 144 beats per minute) to be in the cardio "zone" for an optimal workout. Many cardio machines have sensors that will measure your heart rate, or you can have a fitness trainer or qualified professional calculate your heart rate by taking your pulse from the carotid artery of your neck.

Nutrition Tips and Food Management

Now, one more thing, before we get into the exercises for those problem areas, it's important to talk about your food intake. I always say that about 70% of getting into good shape and being healthy is food management. You can exercise until "the cows come home," but your efforts could be completely erased and nullified by the choices you make on meals and snacks.

What I've learned throughout many years as a health and fitness coach is that if you think you are doing a good job on your food management, you are not. If you think you are doing a great job on your food management, you are only doing a decent job. And, if you think you are doing perfect, you are probably only doing a fairly good job. That's how tough it is to eat properly. Over the past 25-or-so years, portion sizes have gone up something like 600%. Americans eat about 100 pounds more food a year than we did back then. There are more fast food chains and convenience stores all around us, filled with unhealthy and processed foods. We now consume roughly 20% of our daily calories through sugary and fatty beverages (think sodas and Starbucks' white chocolate, mocha-type lattes with whipped cream). All the extra energy from these calories just gets stored as fat in our bodies, because we are also more sedentary.

Creating a perfect storm for overweight and obesity, we work longer hours these days, and commute times are longer than they were 20 years ago. The average American watches around five hours of TV per day. That's not including time on the Internet, surfing the web or watching on-line TV shows or movies, or playing on your smart phone and/or tablet. So, unless you have mastered the art of food management, you risk not burning off enough extra calories to make a substantial impact in your fitness goals. You must become the master of your food and beverage intake.

It's funny, but when you do an on-line search for "diets," you get about 40 million results. I wonder why with that much information right at our fingertips, our fingertips still choose to reach for cookies or pizza?! Over the years I've had clients ask me about crazy diets that involve no carbs, no white foods, higher protein, no fruits or veggies (c'mon does that really sound humanly healthy?), liquids only, raw food only, no eating after 6pm, eating according to your blood type, drinking some type of mother's milk (whose mother I have no idea), eating meat only when the moon is full (okay, not true, but you get the idea). I usually say to them it doesn't have to be rocket science, just stick to the basics and don't over-think it.

Have you ever travelled to another country and wondered why all the people look so thin and still eat normal food, and have dessert? When I went to Paris and observed all the locals still eating their desserts and bread while remaining overall pretty thin-bodied, I observed it's because they eat normal portions and they don't eat very many processed foods. Most things are fresh baked and prepared daily. They probably walk around a lot more than we do here in the States, burning more calories, but I bet they don't have as many gyms as we do. So in regards to dieting, here's one basic down-to-earth strategy: Just focus on what I call your PP (gotcha! No, not that one!): PORTIONS & PROCESSED.

Portions

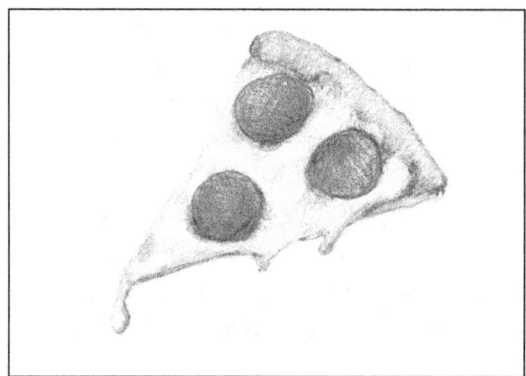

As I mentioned, food portion sizes have gone up drastically in the past few decades. Our bodies just don't require that amount of extra stored energy per meal or snack (which ultimately gets turned into fat on your body). Even if you're eating an organic grilled range free humane certified piece of chicken breast, if it's too large a portion it's just going to get stored as fat.

C'mon, we're not running from Saber Toothed tigers anymore or walking a hundred miles every day, searching for food sources. We're usually stuck in traffic, or lying on the couch, flipping through our 500 cable or satellite channels on our TV's, and/or sitting in front of a computer screen with internet paralysis. Folks, we act like we're pigs at a trough when food is around; we have to remember that food is simply fuel for our bodies and minds.

When you are getting ready to eat, you gotta ask yourself, "Why am I eating this meal?" Is it to provide energy for your work day ahead? Is it to recover after a tough workout? Is it so you have antioxidants to fight off free radicals? Is it for the fiber to help clear out the cholesterol in your body? Whatever the case, each meal and snack you eat should have meaning attached to it.

If you're constantly over-eating and over-indulging, try these tips:

> When you are hungry, wait 10 minutes before eating and then chew your food slowly. It takes 20 minutes for your mind to tell your stomach you are full.

> Drink a glass of water before eating to make you feel fuller.

> Eat foods that are less calorie-dense (i.e. fruits, vegetables).

> Don't eat 1/4 of whatever is on your plate. "Save that for the Devil," as they say.

> Don't keep junk food in the house/apartment. This is a rule that I live by. Most cravings aren't strong enough to make you get in the car and drive down to the store to pick up some junk food. So, if it's not in the house/apartment, then you won't have it. And, by George, amazingly, you'll be thinner and leaner in no time!

In regards to portions, a very simple and easy way to stay on track with your food portions is by using the "eyeball method" to compare proper portion sizes to something that you are familiar with, like a computer mouse or a set of dice.

Familiarize yourself with these and for the rest of your life you'll never have to guess again:

Meat

> 3 ounces of meat: deck of cards or palm of your hand without your fingers

Breads, cereals, rice and pasta

> An average bagel: a hockey puck

> A medium potato: a computer mouse

> 1 cup of rice or pasta: size of your fist

> 1 cup dried cereal: a large handful

Dairy

> 1-1/2 ounces natural cheese: 4 dice

Fats, Oils and Sweets

> 1/2 cup of ice cream: a tennis ball

> 1 teaspoon butter, salad dressing, peanut butter or mayonnaise: one die (dice)

FYI: one tablespoon = 3 teaspoons

Fruit

> 1 medium fruit: a tennis ball

> 1 cup of fruit: a baseball

> 1/2 cup chopped fruit: 15 marbles

Vegetables

> 1 cup lettuce: 4 leaves

> 1 cup vegetables (chopped): a fist

> 1.2 cup vegetables (chopped): light bulb

Processed Foods

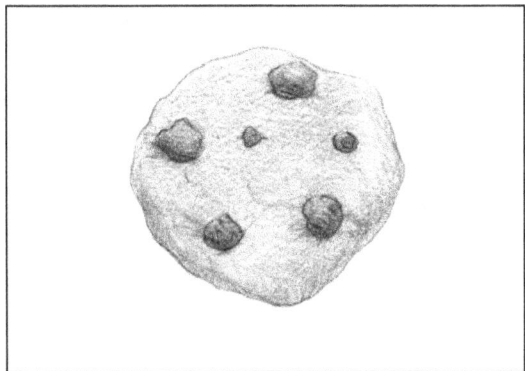

Cheap to manufacture, easy, quick and addictive to eat, but causing disease, depression and obesity like nobody's business. Wean yourself off of eating processed foods and you'll look and feel awesome! Here's how: Start by choosing one day a week where you have absolutely no processed foods. Maybe it would be easier to do it on a weekend if you are less busy and stressed. Remember, only wholesome, natural foods with no extra additives, hormones, or ingredients you can't pronounce. At the end of the day, make it a point to write down how you feel. Do you have more energy? Are you more focused? Do you have less heartburn? Then the next morning, make it a point to document how you feel when you wake up. Are you more alert? Are you more energized? Are you ready to seize the day?

After you have weaned yourself completely off of processed foods, one day a week for 4 weeks in a row, then try to add another day of the week where you are processed-foods free. Yep, that's two complete days per week. You can do it! Keep a journal of how you feel each day. Also, be alert as to how other things in your life might be changing. Are people around you treating you better? Are you more effective and efficient at work? Are you accomplishing more in your personal and professional life? Do you have a more positive attitude in general?

Keep progressing by adding in an additional day of the week that you are processed-foods free. You will be amazed at how your body starts changing for the better. You'll even notice your joints feeling better and having more range of motion! Our body just wasn't meant to have all that crap in it, it doesn't know what to do with it, so it builds up as fat and/or becomes a breeding ground for cancer cells. As they say in Costa Rica, "Pura Vida," which means live the "Pure Life." You'll virtually become a different person without processed foods and experience what the Ticos (local Costa Ricans) mean by that phrase.

Did you know? In the 1960's food manufacturers began using High Fructose Corn Syrup (HFCS) to sweeten foods because it was cheap to use. Since then, as the usage of this sweetener has increased, so has the obesity rate in the USA. HFCS contains elements that inhibit insulin from being released to lower our blood sugar levels. Bottom line, that's real bad.

So remember, if you don't approach your food management with complete urgency, dedication and focus, you absolutely will not succeed in your fitness goals. I came across a poster once that sums it all up, "Anyone can work out for an hour, but to control what goes on your plate the other 23 hours…that's the hard work." Chew on that!

If you are looking to bulk up after the fat loss and build bigger muscles, you may be wondering about consuming extra protein. The RDA (Recommended Daily Allowance) for the general public is 0.8 grams of protein per kilogram of weight. However, there's no RDI for protein intake for athletes. The International Society of Sports Nutrition suggests exercising individuals' protein intake should be between 1.4 and 2.0 g/kg/day, depending on type of exercise and intensity, and a few other factors. While I'm not a nutritionist, I tend to pick a mid-way point for my clients between the general public and exercising individuals' guidelines for daily protein intake, so about 1.4 grams per kilogram of body weight (1 kilogram = 2.2 pounds). Now do the math for your weight. If you weigh 175 pounds, that's roughly 112 grams of protein per day.

It's important to not go too crazy consuming protein powders and shakes though. Consuming high amounts of protein can have some adverse effects, and may not really improve your strength or endurance. You need to understand that the amount of amino acids absorbed from the protein in your gastrointestinal tract is limited, and does have a cut-off point. So those protein powders touting 75 grams per serving, trying to convince you they will make you stronger, is malarkey. Also, high protein diets exceed the liver's capability to convert excess nitrogen to urea. So you must be careful to avoid protein toxicity. Finally, any excess protein the body doesn't use is converted to fat anyway.

One last thing before we get to the exercises for your *Beer Belly, Chicken Legs, Wimp Arms, and Man Boobs*: always check with your doctor before you start any new workout or diet program. It's also a good idea to have a certified and experienced fitness trainer to supervise at least your first few workouts to make sure you are using proper form and not risking injury to yourself. And, always warm up properly before starting your program.

So with all of that said, let's get you CUT, COOL, and CONFIDENT! Use those wimp arms, and turn the page now.

Beer Belly

How to get rid of BEER BELLY, also called Pot Belly, Jelly Roll, or Muffin Top. While drinking beer, it can also be caused by screaming, "Get in my belly," whenever you see junk food in front of you.

Even if you don't drink beer, you can easily start to gain body fat in your stomach if you're not careful. That's where men store much of their excess calories. (By the way, if you do drink beer or any type of alcohol, be aware that it's seven empty calories per gram, almost as much as fat, and your body will always use your alcohol stores before your fat stores for energy, thus making it even harder to burn your fat off.) And it's definitely very important to get excess belly fat under control, as excess belly fat in the midsection is linked to a variety of health problems like type-2 diabetes, high blood pressure, and cardiovascular disease.

I always say the belly fat area is like a bad in-law, it's the first to arrive and the last to leave, so stay focused and committed to the following exercises in conjunction with your cardio to get rid of the beer belly, and you'll be on your way to six-pack abs!

Crunch

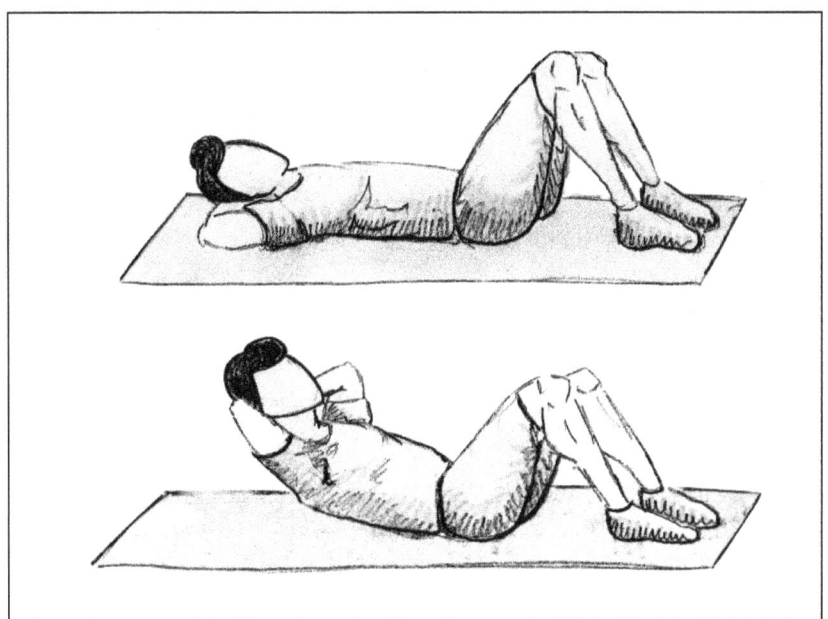

1) Lie on your back, on the floor or a bench, with your knees bent and feet flat on the floor, with your hands behind head. Keep your elbows back and out of sight. Your head should be in a neutral position with a space between your chin and your chest.

2) Leading with the chin and chest towards the ceiling, contract your abdomen and raise your rear shoulders off the floor or the bench.

3) Return back to the original starting position. Remember to keep your head and back in a neutral position.

Bicycles

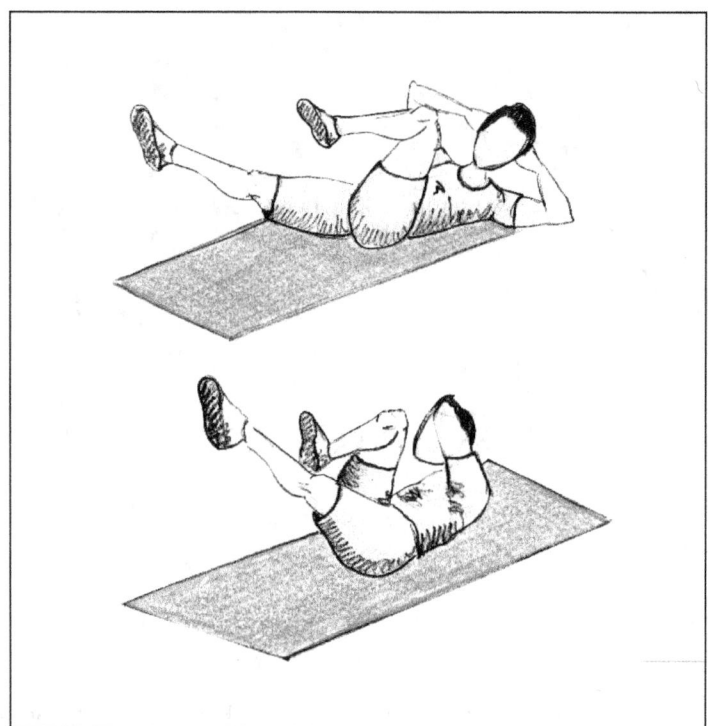

1) Start by lying on your back with your hands clasped behind the back of your neck and your thighs bent 90-degrees at your hip, with feet off the ground and toes pointing towards the ceiling.

2) Simultaneously curl your right shoulder and left knee up and in towards the center of your body until your elbow and knee touch. Extend your leg back and return to the starting position along with your elbow to reset, and then repeat with the other side.

3) Continuously repeat this pattern of kicking your legs in and out while your opposite side elbow moves towards your opposite knee, doing at least 30 repetitions.

Plank Knee-Ins

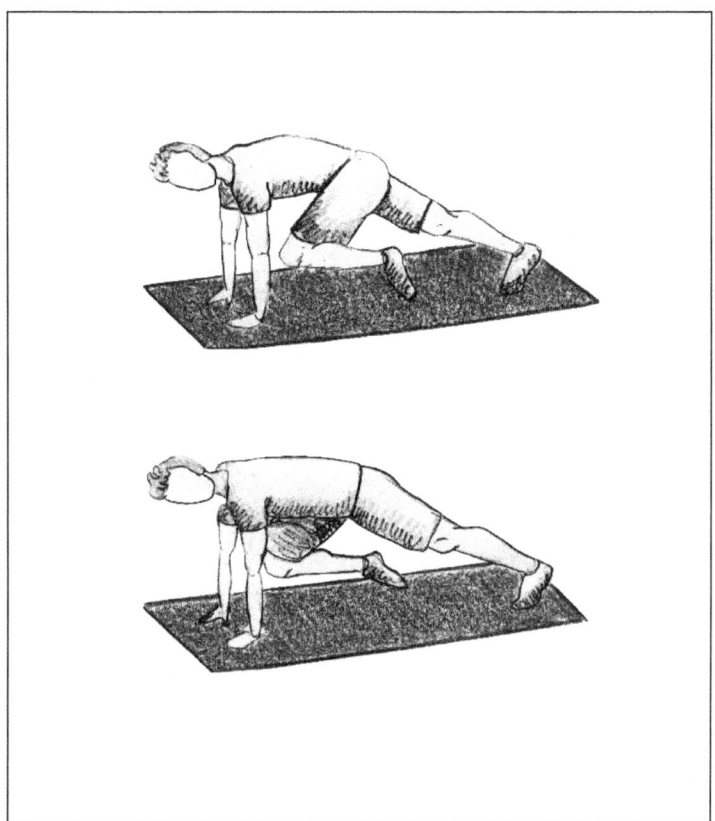

1) Start by getting on your hands and knees in a push-up type position. Raise your knees up off the floor so that only your hands and feet are touching the floor and supporting your weight.

2) Keeping your abs tight and your trunk parallel, bring one knee in towards your chest. Be sure not to raise your butt up too much, putting your body into a "V" shape. Try to keep it straight and parallel to the floor.

3) Return the foot back to the starting position and repeat with the other leg, doing at least 30 repetitions.

Vacuums

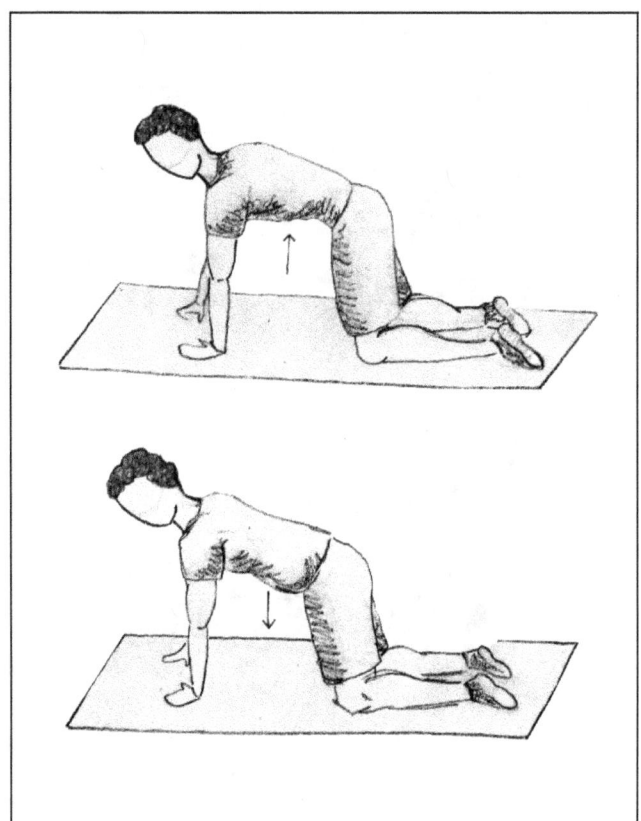

    1) Start by getting on your hands and knees, keeping your head in a neutral position.

    2) In a drawing-in-maneuver, suck your belly button in towards your spine.

    3) Hold for 10 seconds then release.

    4) Repeat for 15 repetitions.

Some additional tips for getting rid of and preventing Beer Belly:

> As mentioned, limit your alcohol intake. The CDC recommends up to one drink per day for women, and two drinks for men. A drink is defined as 12 ounces of beer, or five ounces of wine, or 1.5 ounces or a "shot" of 80-proof distilled spirits or liquor (e.g., gin, rum, vodka, or whiskey).

> Consume no more than 30% of your total daily calories from fat (with no more than 10% coming from the bad fats, which are trans and saturated).

> Consume no more than 100 calories per day from sugar. I'm talking about simple carbohydrates like table sugar, the bad stuff. Always remember, your body needs a certain amount of the good fats like polyunsaturated and monounsaturated, but it doesn't need simple sugar. It's that simple!

Chicken Legs

How to get rid of CHICKEN LEGS, also can be referred to as Toothpick Legs and Skinny Legs

We've all seen the guy in the gym with a big, massive muscular upper body, reminding us of a super hero, but then one glance below the waist reveals a horrible epidemic amongst gym rat types - chicken legs. How can some guys be so impressive and intimidating from the waist up, yet so weak and weary-looking from the waist down? Most skinny legs can be attributed to simple neglect.

In particular, the back of your leg between your butt and knees, which is called the hamstring muscle group, is two-thirds of your leg muscles. So it's very important to focus on building up those muscles to change the appearance of your lower body. And, of course, your quads, which are the front part of your leg between your groin and knees, complete the puzzle.

To build up your leg muscles and say goodbye to those "chicken legs," use heavier weights with fewer repetitions, performing at a slow tempo.

In this book I've concentrated on listing exercises that you can do anywhere, anytime, without the need for expensive equipment or machines. However, for this particular set you will need to find a gym somewhere to use. Pump up with these exercises and watch your legs grow into "tree trunks!"

Lying Hamstring Curl

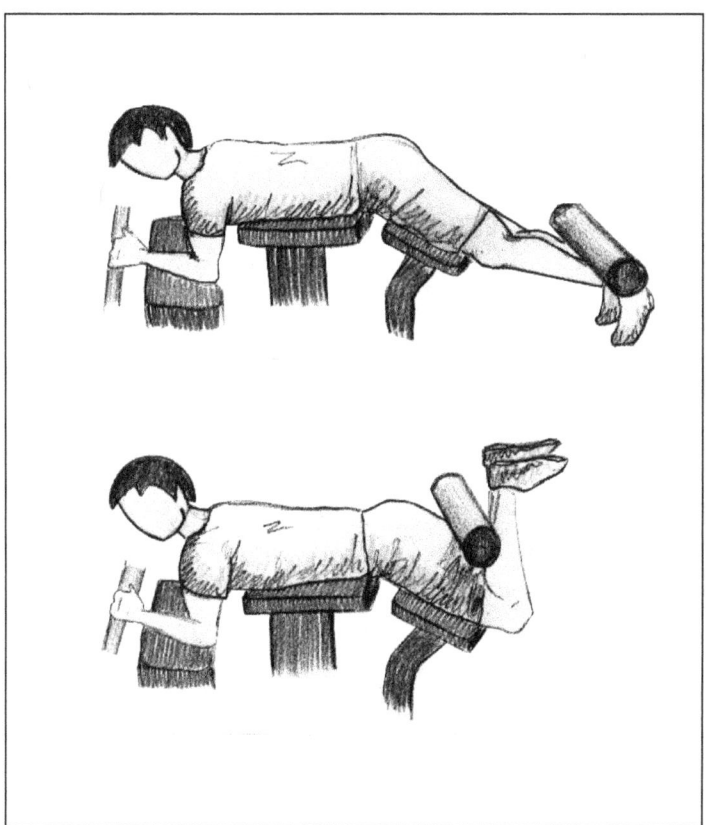

1) Lie face down on a leg curl machine bench with the pad/lever arm adjusted to fit behind your ankles. If the machine does not angle your upper torso downward, you can place a pillow underneath your stomach.

2) Position your knees below the bottom edge of the bench or pad so that they are free to move and not inhibited by the bench. Your legs should be straight and hands grasping the handles or side of the bench.

3) Raise the lever arm by flexing at the knees (curling up) just past 90 degrees.

4) Return back down to the starting position.

5) Remember to keep your hips in contact with the bench at all times. Do not hyperextend your lower back (excessive inward curve) during the movement.

One-Leg-45-Degree Leg Press

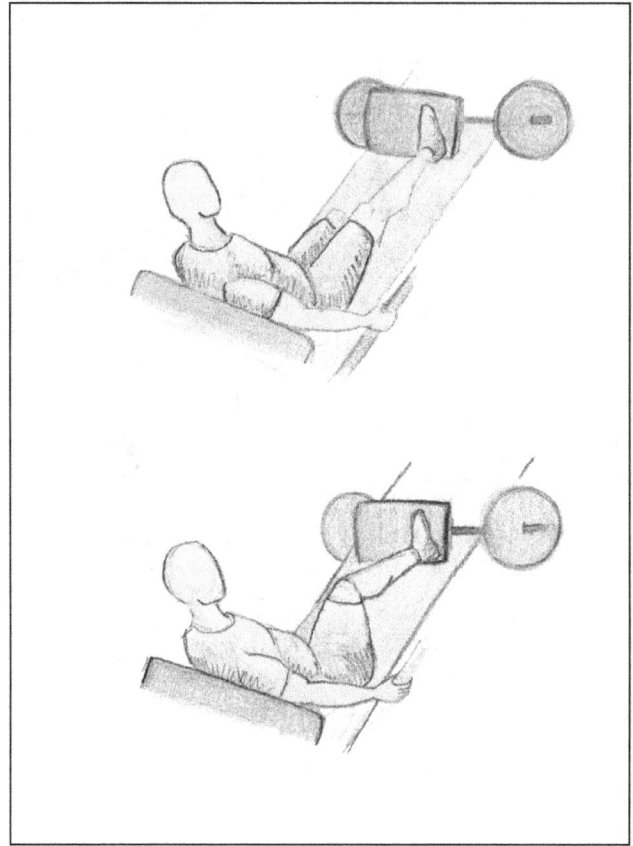

1) Sit in the machine and place one foot onto the footplate, positioned off-center toward the side of whichever leg you are using.

2) Bend your knee and lower the sled down until your knee is bent to about 90 degrees.

3) Press your leg back up to full extension and repeat. Remember to do both legs!

Barbell Squat

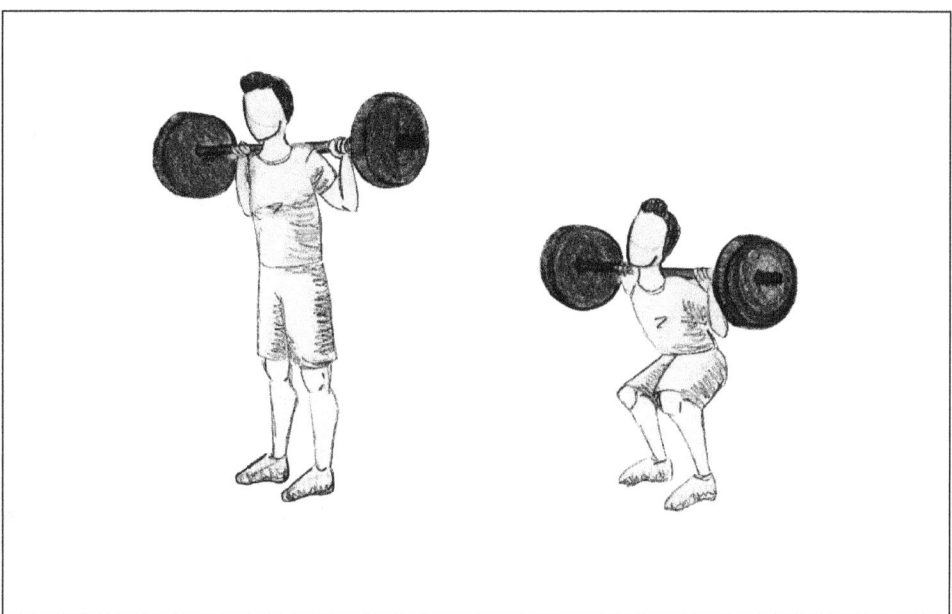

1) Grasp the bar with an overhand grip (palms forward) and slightly wider than hip-width apart. Step under the bar and position the bar across the posterior (rear) deltoids (shoulders) at the middle of your trapezius muscles (shoulder shrugging muscles). DO NOT rest the bar on your actual neck. Lift your elbows up, pull your shoulder blades together, and lift your chest up to create a "shelf" for the bar.

2) Using your legs, remove the bar from the rack. Stand with your feet slighter wider than hip-width apart. Your back should be straight, in a neutral position.

3) Lower your body by flexing at the hips and knees. Your upper body can flex forward at the hips just slightly (~5°) during the movement. Be sure to "sit back" so that your knees stay over your feet.

4) Once your thighs are parallel to floor, return back up to the starting position.

5) Remember to keep your head and back straight in a neutral position - hyperextension or flexion may cause injury. Keep the weight over the middle of your foot and heel, not your toes.

6) DO NOT allow your knees to go past the big toe or deviate medially (inward) or laterally (outward) throughout the movement. Keep your abdominals tight throughout the exercise by drawing your stomach in towards your spine.

Single Leg Dumbbell Calf Raise

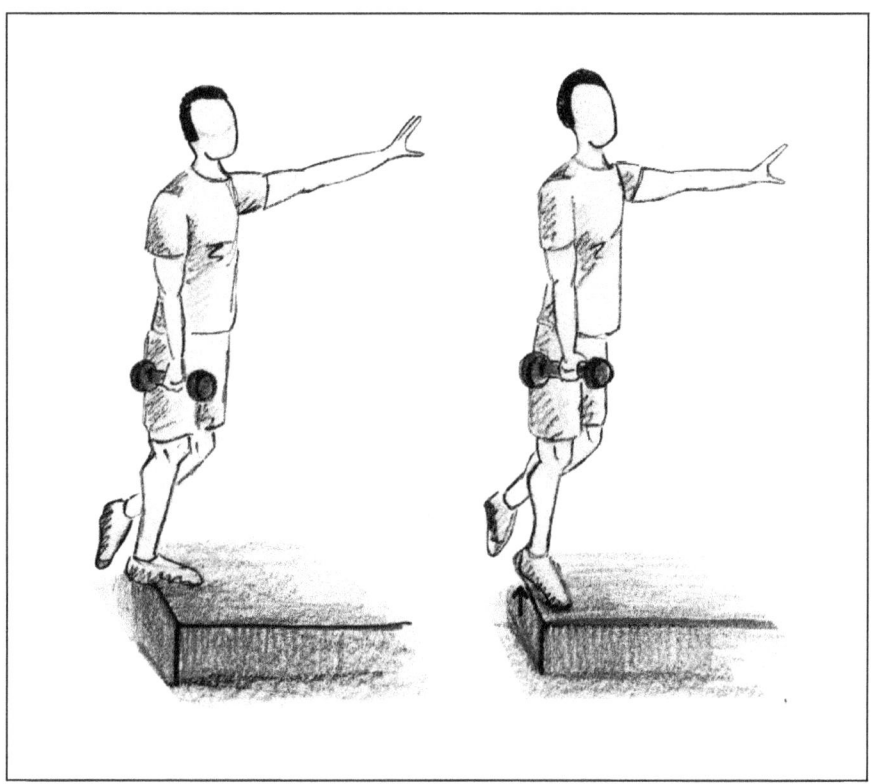

1) Stand with your feet hip-width apart on the edge of a step, with the ball of one foot on the step and your heel hanging over the edge. Raise your other leg back, so that foot isn't on the step. Hold a dumbbell in your hand on the same side as the foot that is on the step. Secure and balance yourself by holding onto a fixed, stationary object with your free hand.

2) Contract your calf by pushing off the ball of your foot to raise your heel up in the air (standing on toes).

3) Lower your heel and repeat.

4) Keep your knee slightly bent throughout the movement to prevent any knee strain.

5) Repeat with the other leg after completing the prescribed repetitions.

Some additional tips on preventing and curing "Chicken Legs":

> Weekly cardio is very important to heart health, weight loss, and positive outlook; however, excessive running, jogging, biking, etc. can be counterproductive to building muscle mass and bulking-up in your legs. It will generally thin and tone your leg muscles. Balance your cardio with leg resistance training to keep your muscle growth optimized.

> As I mentioned, perform your leg routine with heavier weights, doing fewer repetitions, and using a slow tempo. You'll really feel the burn, the lactic acid build-up, and the growth happening.

> Get a good quality night's sleep after an intense weightlifting session. Your muscles will repair themselves and grow while you are sleeping. A lack of sleep throws all your hormone levels off balance, such as testosterone and growth hormones, thus preventing optimal muscle tissue growth. At least 7.5 hours of sleep is recommended!

Wimp Arms

How to get rid of WIMP ARMS, also known as Tyrannosaurus Rex Arms and Weakling Arms.

Some might argue that since the beginning of time, the true measure of a man's brute force and masculinity is measured by only one thing – no, not that! His arms! Turn of the century circus-type pioneering bodybuilder Eugene Sandow developed his arms to amazed onlookers, and Arnold Schwarzenegger flexed his 22-inch arms to win seven Mr. Olympia titles, and children are always dazzled by the size of their dad's or uncle's arms.

So if you have wimp arms, the first thing to take note of is that it really isn't just about the bicep (the front of your arm), because the triceps (the back of your arm) is two-thirds of your arm's muscle. So doing endless sets of barbell curls in the gym ain't gonna get you into the "gun" show.

Do these arm exercises three times per week, and feel your arm sleeves on your shirts start to feel tighter like the Incredible Hulk!

Triceps Bench Dip

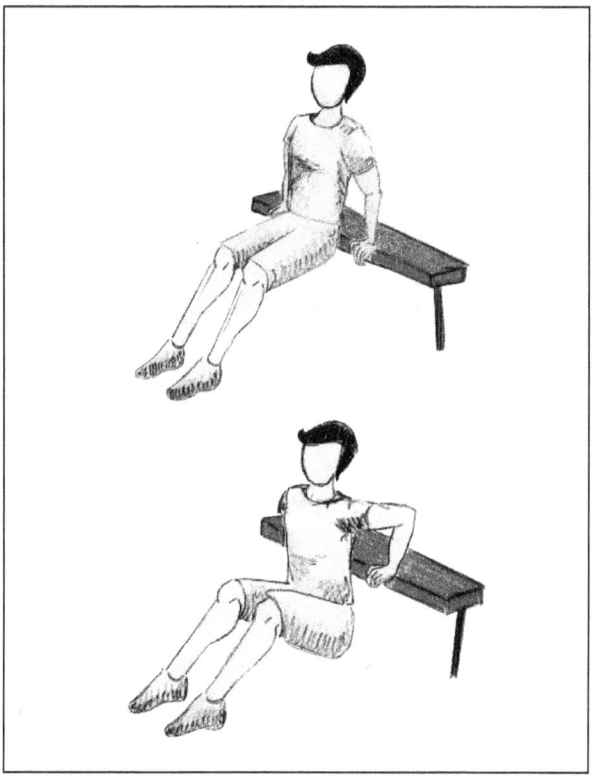

1) Start by placing your hands on a bench or chair and your feet on the ground with your legs bent just slightly.

2) Lower yourself down until your arms are bent to about 90 degrees.

3) Return to the starting position and repeat three sets of 15 repetitions.

Skull Crushers

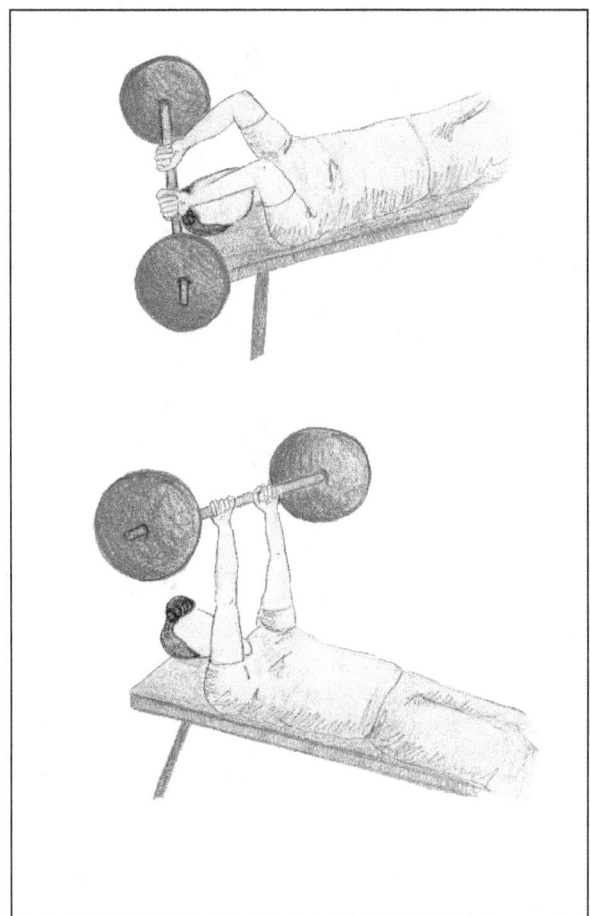

1) Start by lying on a bench and holding a barbell above your chest with your arms straight. Hands should have a medium wide grip, about shoulder width apart.

2) Without moving your shoulders, bend your elbows so that the bar comes down to your forehead level.

3) Stop the bar just before it gets to your forehead and then extend your arms back up to the starting position.

4) Do three sets of 15 repetitions with a moderate weight.

Diamond Pushups

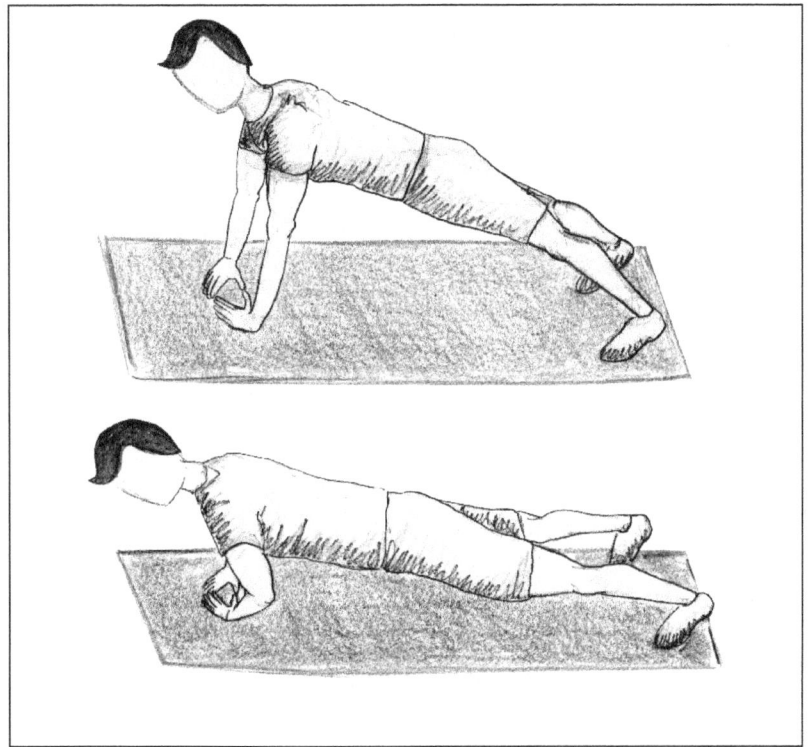

1) Lie face down on the floor and place your hands in the center of your chest, forming a triangle shape with your index fingers and thumbs. Feet should be at hip width with toes on the floor.

2) Extend your elbows and raise your body off the floor.

3) Lower your entire body (legs, hips, trunk, and head) three to seven inches from the floor.

4) Return to the starting position by extending at the elbows and pushing your body up.

5) Remember to keep your body and head in a neutral position, don't raise your hips/butt up too high or droop too low, and never lock the elbows.

Dumbbell Curl (Two Arms)

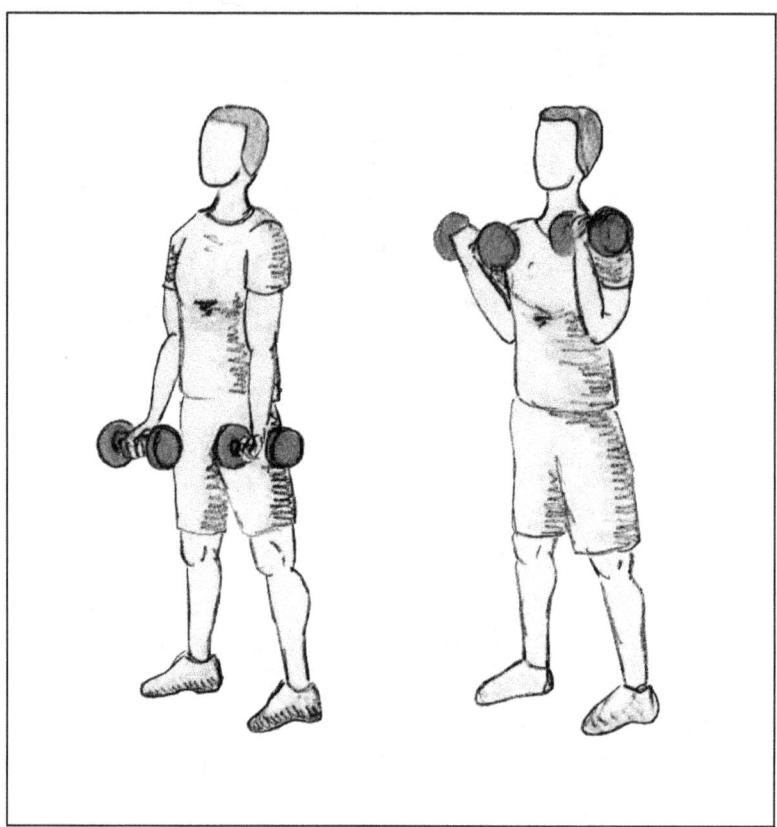

1) Stand with your feet shoulder width apart and knees slightly bent, or sit in an upright position on a bench or stability ball.

2) Grasp dumbbells with an underhand grip (palms facing forward) and allow your arms to hang down at your sides. Your elbows should be close to your sides.

3) Curl the dumbbells up to approximately shoulder level. Keep your elbows close to your sides throughout the movement. Don't arch your back.

4) Return back down to the starting position.

5) During the movement, your shoulders should be stabilized by squeezing your shoulder blades together slightly, only your elbow joint should be moving.

Some additional tips on reducing and getting rid of "Wimp Arms":

>   Remember that anytime you do chest exercises you work the triceps, and anytime you do back exercises you work the biceps. So, in order not to over train the arms, do not do chest and triceps on consecutive days, and do not do back and biceps on consecutive days. You'll need a day's rest to help the arm muscles grow.

>   Exercise machines are great, but don't rely on them too much because they have a fixed range of motion and your body memorizes that range and adapts quickly. Free weights and manual resistance are always the best choices to get those arms big.

Man Boobs

How to get rid of MAN BOOBS, also known as Moobs and Chest Sag

Man Boobs - it's the excess fat stored in the chest on some guys. They droop a little and can jiggle with sudden movements. You may remember that classic Seinfeld episode, "The Mansierre," where Kramer developed a bra for guys (The Bro) who were suffering from a little too much "extra luggage on the top floor." Sometimes they are caused by a hormonal imbalance, a medical condition called "gynecomastia" (see a doctor if you think this is the cause), but most times it's just where your body happens to be storing fat.

Now, I always preach that you can't "spot-reduce" fat and that you will need to eat healthier and exercise more to reduce the total fat percentage in your body. Then and only then will the man boobs start to decrease in size. But it is important to do strength training exercises for your pectoralis muscles (chest muscles) to help shape them into a firm and tight size that you can be proud of when you're at the beach with your shirt off. (And wearing a "Bro" is so uncomfortable when sand gets inside of it.)

Here are some exercises you can do three times per week to target those Man Boobs.

Standard Push-Up

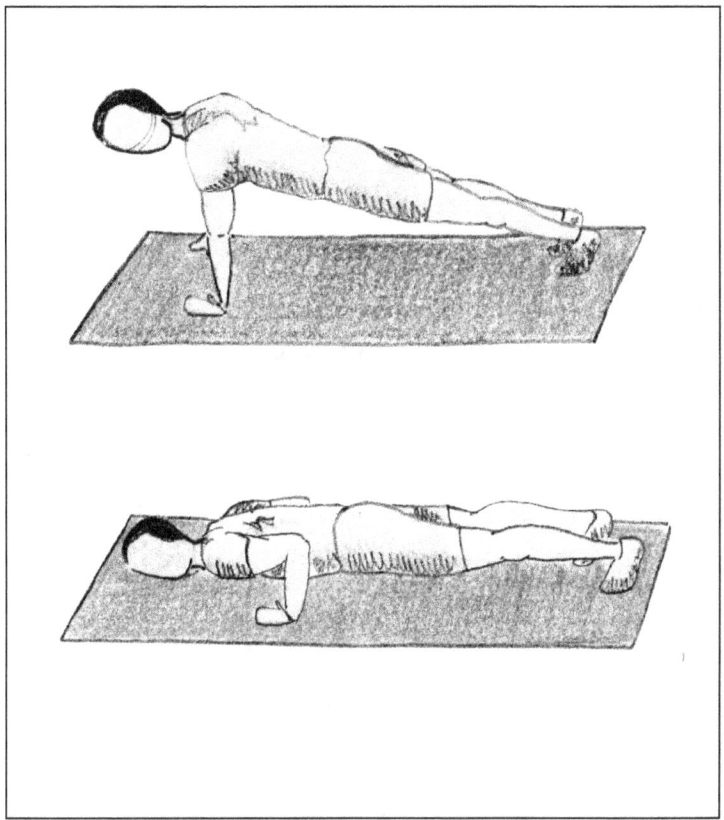

1) Lie face down on the floor with hands palms down, fingers pointing straight ahead, and thumbs lined up at your nipple line.

2) Place your hands slightly wider than shoulder width, and your feet at hip width, with your toes on the floor.

3) Extend your elbows and lift your body off of the floor.

4) Lower your entire body (legs, hips, trunk, and head) 3-6 inches from the floor.

5) Return to the starting position by extending at the elbows and pushing your body up.

6) Remember to keep your head and trunk stabilized in a neutral position and draw your naval into your spine (engage the core). Never fully lock out your elbows, and avoid hyperextension of your low back.

Alternating Dumbbell Bench Press

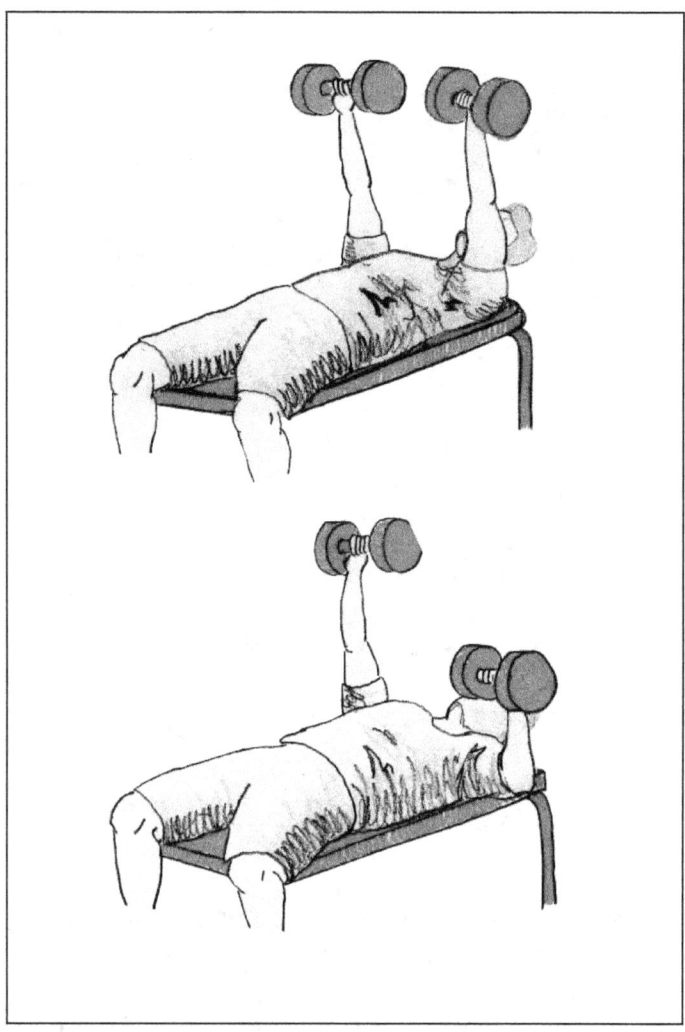

1) Sit in an upright position on a flat bench with a dumbbell in each hand. (You can rest one dumbbell on each thigh.)

2) Lie on your back and bring the dumbbell to your shoulders. Press one dumbbell up directly above the chest with your palm facing forward.

3) Lower that dumbbell all the way down until it's at chest level, keeping your forearms perpendicular to the floor.

4) Then press up with the other arm.

5) Remember to keep both feet flat on the floor at all times and keep your lower back in a neutral position. Hyperextension or arching of the back may cause injury. Never lock out your elbows.

Band Chest Press on Ball

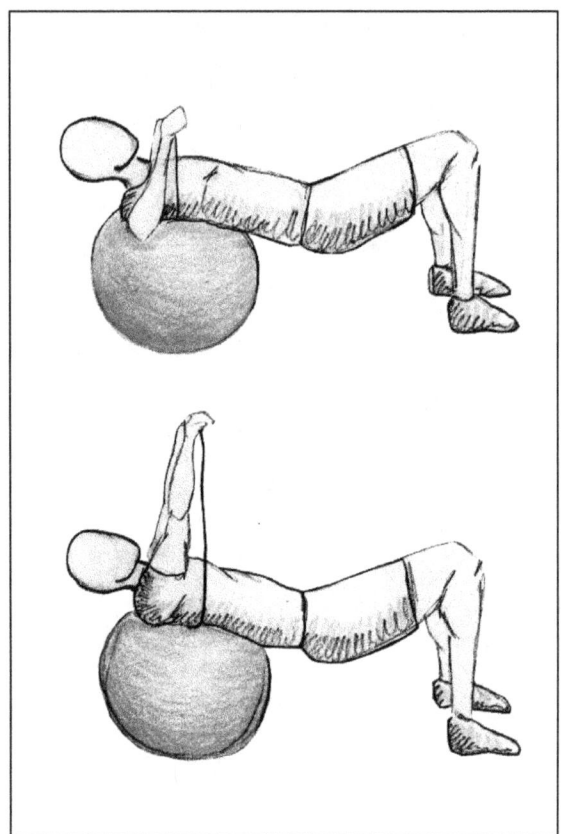

     1) Lie on your back on a Swiss Ball (Resisto-Ball) with your feet firmly on the floor, keeping your hips up and core engaged with a fitness band (tubing) secured under the ball. You can also secure the band under your back, if it is short.

     2) With your arms extended above your chest, slowly bring them down until your hands are at chest level. Keep your forearms perpendicular to the floor and your elbows out just a little bit from your body.

     3) Once your hands reach chest level, press up and return to the starting position and repeat.

Some additional tips for preventing and getting rid of "Man Boobs":

> Droopy shoulders and bad posture can enhance the effects of Man Boobs, so be sure to always include exercises that will strengthen your posture muscles in order to draw your chest out and shoulders back. Good exercises are those for your rear deltoids (shoulders) and your trapezius (traps) muscles. Some examples would include bent over dumbbell rear deltoid lateral raises and shoulder shrugs (either with dumbbells or barbell).

> Other great activities that can help to reduce those Man Boobs include boxing, swimming, and playing the accordion. (And here's a worthless trivia tidbit: 1900-1960 was often referred to as the Golden Age of the Accordion.)

Staying Motivated and Engaged

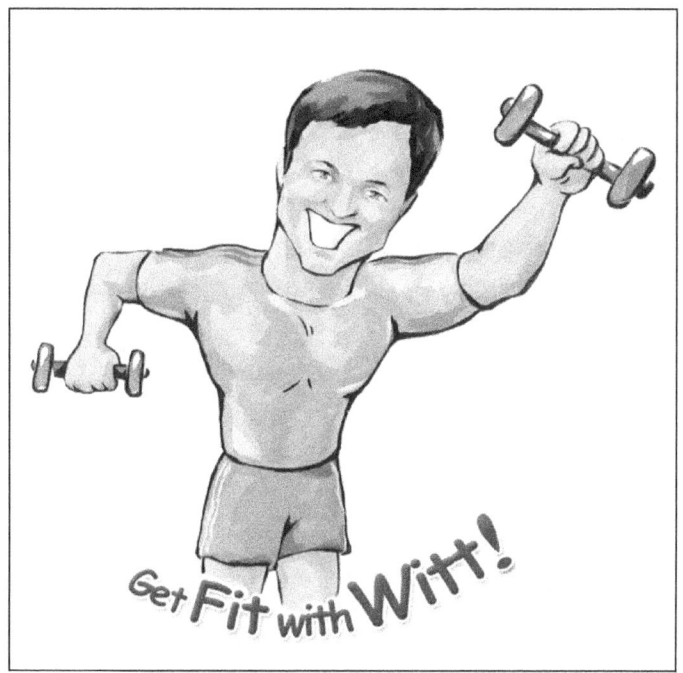

There are going to be a lot of distractions, obstacles, and barriers to your success along the way when getting rid of Beer Belly, Chicken Legs, Wimp Arms, and Man Boobs, and more. So when you "fall off the wagon," here's how to pick yourself back up and resume your forward momentum, taking charge of your health and wellness.

Forget Perfection

First of all, always remember that you are not perfect, and that even fitness professionals like me have bad days where we slip on our diet or our exercise. The most important thing to do is simply "take two." Remember how I talked about this being the movie of your life, starring YOU and also directed by YOU? So if you slip up and overeat or skip a workout session, just remember your movie has a big budget and you can re-shoot the scene the next day for a second take. Don't beat yourself up, just take "action" and get back in the scene and give an award winning performance the next day.

Look Beyond the Cosmetic Effects

Second, go beyond the cosmetic benefits of exercising and eating right. About two weeks into your program, start to write down and record other benefits such as, "feel more flexible," or, "more energy and endurance at work," or even, "sleeping better now." After adopting a healthier lifestyle, the benefits to you will be numerous, each one building on a previous benefit until pretty soon it's a snowball effect of good things.

Here are just some of the things I've heard over the years from my clients after they've taken charge of their health and wellness:

- "Less stiffness and pain in joints"
- "Better mental focus and clarity"
- "Able to manage stressors better"
- "Stronger and more flexible"
- "I'm simply happier"
- "Improvement in biomarkers"
- "Better range of motion"
- "Less headaches"
- "Better eyesight"
- "More self confidence"
- "Improved bone density"
- "Easier pregnancy and birth"
- "Reduction in T-cell count"
- "Weight loss"
- "Body fat loss"
- "Improved sport performance"
- "Cure diabetes"
- "Better balance "
- "Less heartburn and acid reflux"
- "Drink less alcohol"
- "Less sickness with flu and colds "
- "Breathe easier"
- "More sociable"
- "Quality time with my children"
- "Able to volunteer more"
- "More spiritual"
- "Stronger faith"
- "Urge to pursue my dreams"

And the list goes on and on and on and on and on and on! Kind of seems too good to be true, doesn't it? Well, it isn't. I've seen and witnessed all this for the past 10 years through my business, GetFitwithWitt.com.

Some other benefits are: the longer you remain consistent with maintaining an exercise program and good eating habits, the more efficient your body will become at burning off its fat stores for an energy source during exercise. Your body relies on stored carbohydrates (glycogen stored in the body) for energy, too, especially for more intense, shorter-duration exercises. Lower intensity, longer-duration exercises tend to utilize more of your fat stores for energy, so here you can see how jogging, hiking, or biking can be a great way to start to train your body to use fat for fuel. Once that starts happening, when you do more intense shorter-duration workouts such as resistance training, your body becomes better at switching over to fat for fuel.

Also, as we age our muscle mass starts to decrease, which makes our metabolism slow down (metabolism is our body's ability to convert food and other substances into energy, essentially its calorie burning ability). In particular, this becomes a real issue for people over the age of 50. Strength and resistance type of exercises help to retain as much of your muscle mass as possible, therefore keeping your metabolism elevated. Always remember a pound of fat on your body only burns about 2 to 3 calories per day, whereas a pound of lean skeletal muscle burns roughly 50 calories per day. Can you see the difference it can make as you replace your body fat with lean skeletal muscle tissue? Your body becomes a lean, mean calorie burning machine, even while you are watching TV and sleeping!

Putting It All Together

So there you have it, folks, a way to take charge of your health and well being while also getting rid of those pesky problem areas on your body, to look and feel your best every single day. I implore you to, "Stop Making Excuses, Focus, and Do Something About It." SMEFADSAI, SMEFADSAI, SMEFADSAI!!

What are you going to do tomorrow to strengthen your emotional intelligence? Create a network of support and friends? How about your faith in fitness? And what about your ability to just immerse yourself into this and get a little bit crazy?

Stay focused on all of these by keeping a journal highlighting each day's SMEDFADSAI and the benefits you are starting to realize from your exercise and diet program. Perhaps a blog would be ideal for you, or a daily status update on Facebook or Twitter. Organize your life from here on out, to keep you focused, informed, and motivated to becoming the real YOU.

The fitness road ahead isn't going to be easy, there are going to be barriers and obstacles that you will need to overcome and get past. One of biggest challenges I hear from people these days is that they think they don't have TIME. The bottom line on this one, you absolutely have to make and carve out the time somehow. This is your life, your health, your wellness, and your happiness. You have to be able to find at least 30 minutes a day for moderate to strenuous physical activity. Get up earlier, do two 15-minute exercise sessions throughout the day, cut down on TV and computer time in order to fit in an exercise session, etc. The TIME thing can't be an excuse; it's just not acceptable.

Another big obstacle I see clients struggle with is food management. Again, this is in my opinion 70% of becoming healthy and in shape. Don't let it discourage you if you fall off track one day and overeat. Just resume again on your path to health and wellness and try to counter the bad day by eating extra good foods the next day. It's a constant balancing act with food, nobody eats perfectly, but as long as you counter any bad behaviors with a resulting extremely good behavior, you should be fine. It's when you stay off course and revert back to a "give up" attitude that you fail to open the door for the real YOU to blossom.

Healthy, Fun and Easy Recipes

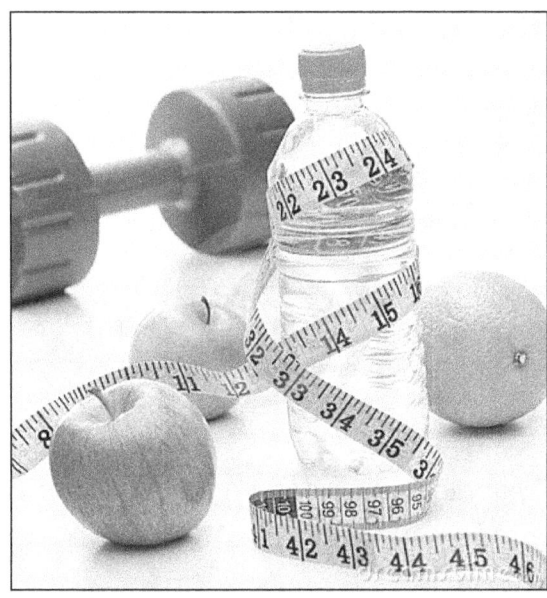

Mojgan's Heirloom Tomato Truffle Salad

Chunks of 2 color tomatoes, chunks of watermelons/any melon (steak thickness cut). Drizzle with nice vinaigrette and truffle oil.

Susan's Hummus Egg Cups

Take a boiled egg, cut in half and ditch the yoke, fill the egg white cups with hummus - a high protein pick me up with very low calories.

Susan's Greek Yogurt/Salsa Dip

Mix one individual size non-fat green yogurt cup with hot/spicy prepared salsa, to taste.

Pair dip with: carrots, sliced Persian cucumbers, or red pepper slices.

You'll get your protein, veggies and spices (good for inflammation).

Anna's Cucumber Soup

(Serves 4)

Ingredients:

1 lb long cucumbers, peeled and coarsely grated
1 garlic clove, crushed
1 tsp ground cumin
2 cups unsweetened natural yogurt
1/2 cup vegetable stock + extra in reserve
Salt
3 tbsp chopped pistachios, for serving
3 tbsp dill sprigs, for serving

Instructions:

Blend cucumber, garlic, cumin and yogurt in a food processor until smooth.

Transfer to a mixing bowl and stir in stock, adding more if soup is too thick. Season to taste.

Cover soup and refrigerate for at least 30 minutes to chill. Serve soup topped with pistachios and dill.

The Get Fit with Witt ! Mid-afternoon Power Punchin' Pick-me-Upper

In a large bowl place:

1 sliced medium banana
1 cup of plain Nonfat Greek Yogurt
2 tablespoons of All-Natural Unsalted Smooth Peanut Butter
1 tablespoon of Raw-Wild Natural Honey

Sprinkle on top (sparingly) some Grape Nuts cereal to give it a crunch.

Annie's Favorite Greek Yogurt Snack

1 carton (6oz) Fahe Greek nonfat yogurt
1 tbspn low calorie fruit jam (25-35 calories)
Handful of raisins, blueberries or diced fresh fruit

1 tbspn chopped or sliced almonds, peanuts, walnuts or pecans

1 tbspn granola

Cinnamon and nutmeg to taste.

First blend yogurt and jam, then add remaining ingredients, and sprinkle the spices on last.

Lifestyle Insights Reports

"It's an Owner's Manual for your Body & Mind"

One of my staple products throughout the years to help people take charge of their health and wellness is my "Lifestyle Insights Report," an owner's manual for your body and mind that you can refer back to for the rest of your life, because it's created for YOU by YOU!

Here's how it works: You'll take a quick 10-minute assessment online, which will generate a customized 18-page report that will pave the way toward your self-discovery. Lifestyle Insights will help you stop stressors before they happen, break bad habits, tap into your personal energy, and get truly motivated to make positive changes in your life. You'll get to know yourself better, understand how your body's inter-related systems affect you, and gain valuable insight into your own unique behavior style. The Lifestyle Insights system will then help you create a 30-day action plan, based on your personal self-discovery process.

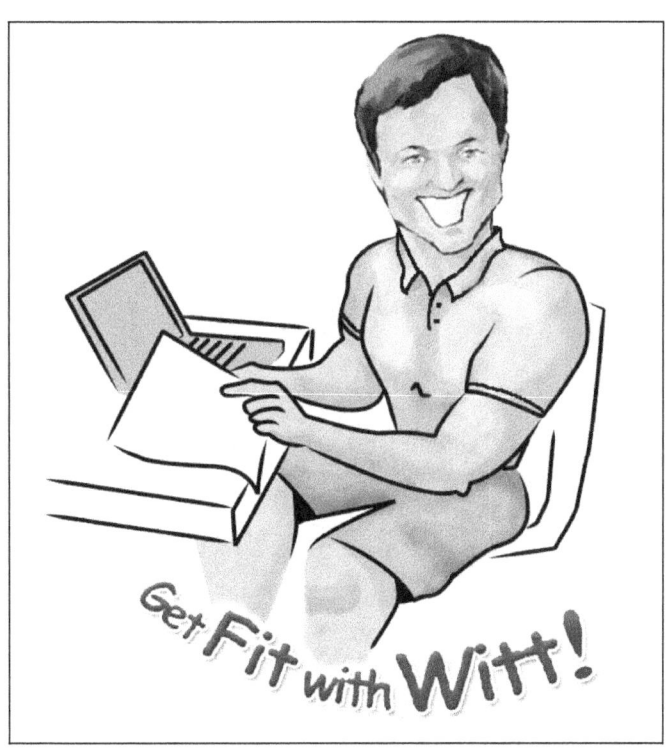

It's important to understand that if your natural and adapted styles don't match, you are probably under too much stress and pressure, by putting your "mask" on every day. With *Lifestyle Insights Reports* you will gain an understanding of your individual style, including insight into your strengths and weaknesses, so that you can reach your full potential.

Order your Lifestyle Insights Report today for only $99 - which includes your Lifestyle Insights Report, Self Guided Workbook, along with additional online tools. As a Professional Certified Behavioral Analyst, I'm personally available to guide you through a 60-minute intensive telephone debriefing session for an additional $59.

You can view a sample report and purchase your *Lifestyle Insights Report* on my website GetFitwithWitt.com or email me directly at Jack@GetFitwithWitt.com.

Special Thanks and Dedication

Kaitlin Howell - for the fun and retro looking illustrations to go along with these books.

Leslie Le Mon - for her coaching and feedback along every step of the way of the journey of writing and publishing my first book(s). Email her at les.lemon.author@gmail.com as she is always happy to consult with writers, first-time or otherwise.

Cherie Higgins - for proofing the book(s).

All my personal fitness training clients throughout the years who would come up to me from time to time and ask me how to get rid of these certain fatty, flabby and out of shape areas on our bodies, and called them by the funny names referenced in the book title. You guys absolutely set the wheels in motion for these books! *Stefanie, Lisa, Ilene & Jim & Sylvia, Alda, Kara & both Davids, Eric, Cookie, Erwin, Mark, Youchanan, Jim, Betsy, Anna, Tanya, Paulina, Selenne, Sonia, Annie!, Kirk, Aliki, Leanne, Jeanne, Jane & Keith, Tony & Lana, Sheila, Gloria, Elizabeth, Lisa, Ellen and Elaine, Lisa and Nancy and Jessica, Jane & Dorain, Susan, Emily, Thang & Nancy, Paul, Lou, David, Sean, Kimberly, Annie, Kevin, Scott, Stacy and Matt, Phil, Elaine (Ink), Stephanie, King, Donna, Michael, Jaime and Jackie, Chris, CherylAnn, Stuart &Robin, Jane & Dorain, MaryLu, Karen & Karen & Andreas, Roz, Ricky, Beneranda, Mayra, Breanna, Sylvia, Mojgan, Patricia, Gina & Dezi & Anna, Bill, Marlene & Chris, Roni and Tess, Stuart & Robyn, Zaven, Justin, Kristie, LuLu, Trudy,* and *Howard.*

Greg Highley - for my personal photographs.

Rony Armas & Agnes Avagyan - for the cartoon Jacks.

Adisorn "Tan" Toonsap - for photo editing.

Carrie Spencer - for Webmastering.

The personal fitness training gyms that I've worked with over the years, including *BodyImage, AtOneFitness, BodyUSA, ShapeIt,* and *Knuckles.*

Some of the other super great fitness trainers I've had the opportunity to work on community and charity projects with over the years – *Nancy Sexton, Steven Greene, Lisa Smith* and *Wendie Wilson.*

NohoArtsDistrict.com - for allowing me the forum to blog and write about fitness and health, and in which I first introduced explanations and exercises for many of these funny named problem body areas.

The *California Jaycees* and the *UCNH Chamber of Commerce* - for invaluable experience helping to build my leadership and business skills, as well as my network of community contacts; many of whom still train with me to this day. And the other community groups I've had the pleasure to build healthy community with, such as *The North Hollywood Rotary, North Hollywood/Studio City Kiwanis, Encino Chamber, North Hollywood High School Key Club* and *NoHo Communications Group*.

One of my very first clients, *Stefanie Ibanez* - for coming up with my business tag line/name: *"Get Fit with Witt!"* Shout it out, people!!

SADA Systems - for developing and managing my website and hosting.

The late *Deby Harper* - for introducing me to *Lifestyle Insights* and helping me personally discover more about myself.

This book is dedicated to one of the most beloved baseball and football little league coaches out of Northeast Ohio; my Dad, *Jack Howard Witt*. He taught us kids to play fair, not to underestimate ourselves or what we could achieve as a team, and to be proud of who we are. RIP, Coach!

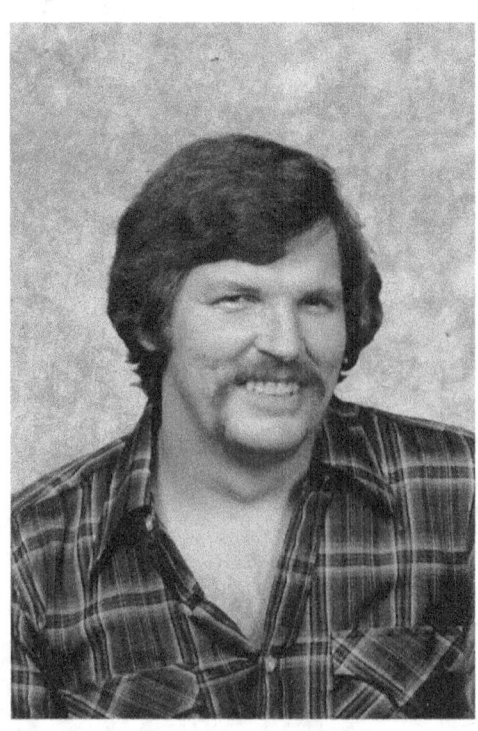

About the Author

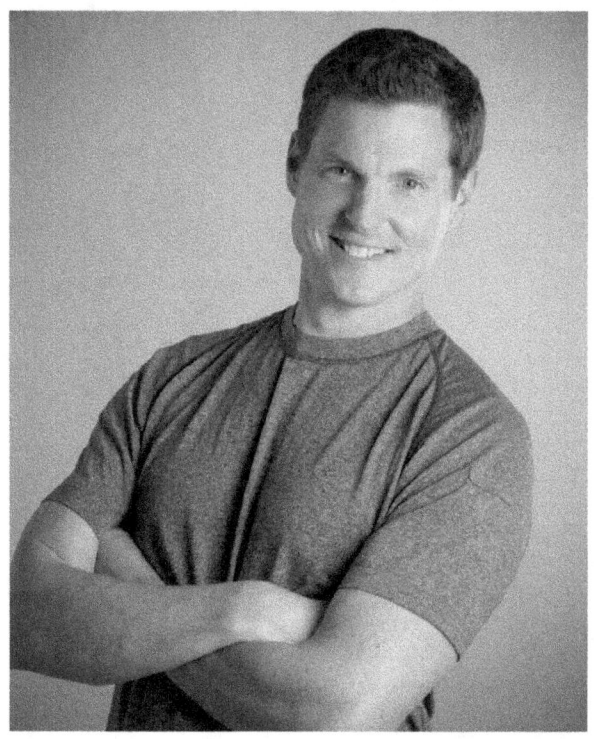

Jack Witt is a health and fitness coach, based out of Los Angeles since 2003. He holds a Master's Degree in Exercise Science, and is a healthy community organizer, serving as past President of the Universal City North Hollywood Jaycees (Junior Chamber) and Chamber of Commerce. His awards include "Outstanding Young Californian", "Angel" and "Small Business of the Year."

He is an NASM Certified Personal Fitness Trainer and TTI Certified Behavioral Analyst. His public speaking and workshop engagements include Los Angeles Unified School District, Social Security Administration, Volunteer League of the San Fernando Valley, and Los Angeles Valley College. Jack has worked with kids, adults and seniors, helping all of them take charge of their health and wellness.

Visit Jack's website at www.GetfitwithWitt.com

Follow Jack on Twitter @GetfitwithWitt

Subscribe to Jack's YouTube Channel at:
http://www.youtube.com/user/getfitwithWitt

Copyrights

All content, illustrations, and photos in *Cut, Cool and Confident: How to get rid of Beer Belly, Chicken Legs, Wimp Arms, and Man Boobs. And much, much more!,* including the cover design; are created by, property of, and copyrighted by Jack Witt © 2013. Healthy Recipe Photo Source: Google Images. Exercise instructions inspired by FitnessGenerator.com.